REGGIE THE GOAT

By Frances Altman

50 Years a Classic

Dedicated to Karen, Allison.
Hannah and all children who enjoy
the antics of a friendly goat.

Registered with Library of Congress 2017
ISBN 9781548165994

Other books by Frances Altman

Escape to Freedom

Spirit Dog

Mr. Umbrella Man, Stories about Inventions

The Something Egg

General Douglas MacArthur, Military Genius

Dwight D. Eisenhower, Crusader for Peace

George Gershwin, Master Composer

Herbert V. Prochnow, Banker

Reggie the Goat

A round shiny quarter tumbled from Gilbert's bank. After it came nickels and dimes and pennies. Gilbert stacked the coins in piles of one dollar each. Then he counted them.   At last he had saved enough to buy a red collar and a warm doghouse.

Now his mother would let him go to the animal shelter and choose a dog as his own pet!

But Gilbert never dreamed there would be so many dogs at the shelter. Dozens and dozens of all kinds of dogs!

Little dogs! Big dogs! Short, fat, tall and lean dogs! Dogs with long velvet ears and dogs with stubby wagging tails! White! Black! Spotted and speckled dogs!

Suddenly Gilbert saw the **one** he wanted! It was all white with a tiny black spot on the tip of each ear.

"I want that one!" he announced decisively.

"What?" The shelter keeper blinked. Still—he had been wanting to find that **goat** a home for a long, long time!

Just to be sure, the keeper asked Gilbert one question.

"Will it be all right with your mother?"

"Oh, she won't mind," Gilbert assured him. "I already have a nice house for him to sleep in."

Without another word the shelter keeper let Gilbert lead the goat away.

"I think I will call you Reggie," Gilbert told his new pet. "Reggie is a very dignified sounding name, don't you think?"

But Reggie **was not** a dignified goat! He was so happy to be out of the shelter that he began to run and jump and frolic in circles.

"Stop! Stop!" shouted Gilbert. But Reggie went right on jumping until his feet were all tangled in the new red leash.

"Reggie, Reggie," scolded Gilbert. "You must learn to walk quietly. See how all the people are walking along the sidewalk."

For a short time Reggie did walk quietly. And Gilbert did not even mind that people were turning their heads to stare as they passed.

Ooops!

A door began to swing open right in front of them.

Gilbert tugged hard on the leash. Reggie jerked harder on the other end. Together they went flying through the door.

"Reggie! This is a bakery!"

It was too late.

Reggie was already nibbling at a large cake in the window. His ears were pointed up. His eyes were shining and his white nose was covered with thick pink frosting.

At that moment the baker saw Reggie!

"Shoo! Shoo!"

He waved his arms wildly at the sight of a goat eating his beautiful cake.

But the baker only made Reggie frolic all the more. In and out behind the counter he trotted. Then back into the baking room he galloped with Gilbert still holding tightly to the leash.

"Stop that goat!' shouted the baker, chasing after them both. "You are ruining my bakery!"

Tins and pans and cookie cutters bounced and clattered to the floor. Great white puffs of flour went rising to the ceiling.

Bang!

Crash!

Thud!

Everywhere Gilbert looked something was going wrong. Gooey icing flooded the cakes and the cookies and even the breads.

The doughnut machine was throwing doughnuts every which way around the room.

At that very moment, another baker happened to open the door.

"What is going on in here?

He was nearly knocked over as Reggie galloped past him with Gilbert close behind.

Out one door!

In another!

"Ahhhhh!

Eckkkkk!"

Ladies screamed as Reggie came bouncing into the discount store.

Sun hats, shoes, and dishes all went toppling to the floor. Once Reggie even looked out the front window and blatted "Naaaa" at all the people out in the street.

Four little hoof prints and a trail of white flour ran everywhere.

Finally, still dragging Gilbert, Reggie trotted out the wide front door and down the street. At the corner he dropped down to rest and watch the cars.

"Oh, Reggie!" He sighed.

"What are we going to do?"

Gilbert threw has arms around Reggie's neck. The goat still had a flowered hat caught between his short horns.

"How will I ever get you home if you keep acting like this? I'm already so tired I can't walk another step!"

But so many people were beginning to gather around them that Gilbert could not rest.

"Come along, Reggie," He tried to coax the goat to his feet. "We must find a way home."

Just then a bus pulled up to the corner.

"May we ride home on your bus?"

Gilbert asked the driver.

"Gracious no!" exclaimed the driver.

"We don't carry goats!"

There was only one thing left to do,

Gilbert decided. He would have to

disguise Reggie so no one would know

he was a goat.

Slowly Reggie and Gilbert walked along as Gilbert tried to think how it could be done. Suddenly he saw a large box that some store had thrown away. And, it was just the right size too.

Gilbert made Reggie jump into the big box. Then he closed the flaps down.

Now there was only one thing wrong. Gilbert could not lift or push or even pull the box one inch.

"Oh, Reggie, what can we do?" cried Gilbert. But Reggie only wanted to crunch on the cardboard flaps.

"Maybe we could put a paper bag over your head."

But when Gilbert found a paper bag on the street and tried it, Reggie's horns popped through.

Next Gilbert paid a quarter for a large shopping bag and tore a hole in the side for Reggie's nose. With another quarter he bought a yard of ribbon and tied the handles around Reggie's neck.

"Taxi! Taxi!" Gilbert called out. "Will you take us home?"

The taxi driver looked very curiously at Reggie with the bag over his head. Then he shrugged.

"Hop in," he said.

Gilbert fell back exhausted against the soft seat. At last they were on their way home.

"Mulberry Road," Gilbert told the driver. Then he closed his eyes to rest.

But Reggie did not want to rest. He craned his bag-covered head over the front seat.

"Naaaaaa! Naaaaaa!" he

blatted

Gilbert's eyes popped open just as

the taxi came to a screeching stop.

"Naaaaaa!"

bleeted Reggie, blinking at the

driver. He had eaten the bottom out of

the shopping bag.

'Get out!" shouted the driver at them both.

"A goat in my taxi! Never! Never! Never!"

Gilbert led Reggie out of the taxi and watched it roar away. Then he looked up at the street sign. They were almost home anyway.

Gilbert left Reggie tied to a tree while he went into the house to find his mother.

"I'm going to put Reggie in his house now," Gilbert told her.

"Hurry right back," she replied "It's nearly time for dinner."

Gilbert led Reggie into the backyard. There stood the trim white doghouse. **But something was wrong.**

First Gilbert looked at the doghouse and then he looked at Reggie. Reggie would **never** be able to get into that house! His legs were too long. His neck was too long. **All of Reggie was too long.**

Gilbert sighed. There was only one other place where he could put Reggie until he figured out what to do. In the basement.

Very quietly Gilbert opened the basement door.

"Shhhh," he whispered to Reggie.

Gilbert hoped Reggie would not be afraid, for it was as dark as night in the basement.

"Tomorrow I will build a bigger house for you. But tonight **please** be very quiet."

Contentedly Reggie lay down by the stairs and closed his eyes. He looked very tired.

Seeing this, Gilbert happily went upstairs where his father and mother were already seated at the table.

Bang!

Bump!

Thud!

"Whatever is that?" asked Gilbert's father.

Bang!

Bump!

Thud!

The sound came again but even louder.

"Something is in the basement," Gilbert's father said.

He picked up a broom and headed for the stairs. Before Gilbert could say one word his father was out of sight.

"Now what can it be?" wondered Gilbert's mother, going down the stairs too.

Gilbert followed slowly behind them. There was no need for him to hurry. He already knew what it was.

"Naaaaaaaa! Naaaaaa! "

From a corner of the room two round white eyes blinked at the three of them.

"Turn on the light!" Ordered Gilbert's father.

"Why, it's a …" He stammered and stopped and began all over again. "It's a goat!"

"A goat?" asked Gilbert's mother in surprise.

"A goat," confirmed Gilbert.

Poor Reggie! This time his feet were tangled in an old pair of boots and a butterfly net had fallen down over his head.

"What is a goat doing in our basement?" asked Gilbert's mother. Then she remembered something.

"Gilbert! Did you bring that goat in here?"

Gilbert slowly nodded.

"But you were going to get a dog," his mother reminded him.

"I thought a goat would be a much better pet," answered Gilbert. Sadly he went over to Reggie and put his arms around his neck.

Gilbert's father put the broom away. Then he, too, went over to Reggie and laid his hand on the goat's head.

"What will we do with a goat? He can't stay here!"

That very night Gilbert's father began telephoning many people that he knew.

He talked to a farmer and to a policeman, to a lawyer and to a man who wrote stories for a newspaper. A photo of Reggie even appeared on an evening television news program.

At last with everyone's help, they were able to find just the right kind of home for Reggie. Where?

The Zoo! A place with trees and grass and where many other kinds of other animals also lived.

When they all arrived at the Zoo, Gilbert's father said: "I guess the city has been a pretty dull place for a goat."

Gilbert's eyes twinkled when he heard this because he was remembering their fast visit to the bakery and the discount store and their ride in the taxi.

"My gracious no!" Gilbert exclaimed. "It's just that there are **too many things for a goat to do in the city!**"

So every Sunday Gilbert, along with many other boys and girls, went to the Zoo to visit Reggie. In fact Reggie was so friendly that he did not have to live in a cage, but could run free all he wished.

In fact, it was not long before Reggie became the official Zoo greeter. That meant that he could wrinkle his nose and go

"Naaaaaaa"

to every person he met!

www.ingramcontent.com/pod-product-compliance
Lightning Source LLC
Chambersburg PA
CBHW061929280526
45787CB00004B/1532